Handy, Healing

TEA TREE OIL

Dr. Joyce Tellier Johnson, ND

© Mind Publishing Inc., 2007

ISBN 978-0978279714

Printed in Canada

Contents

Introduction to Tea Tree Oil

AUSTRALIA, one of the world's most popular travel destinations, has many claims to fame. On the natural health scene one of the most valued exports from "down under" is an essential oil from the Melaleuca alternifolia tree— commonly known as tea tree oil.

Once found only in Southeastern Australia, tea tree oil is fast becoming a global product. There are even plantations springing up in California. The trees grow to a height of approximately 20 feet, and while the whole tree is valued, only the leaves are used to produce the medicinal oil.

The Bundjalong aboriginal people of northern New South Wales Australia have known of the medicinal properties of this tree for many centuries, but it wasn't until 1770 that the Western world named it "tea tree." Captain James Cook found its aromatic leaves an enjoyable substitute for real tea when he arrived in New South Wales. Gradually settlers, observing the natives, began to use the leaves and volatile oil obtained from them in the treatment of cuts, abrasions, burns, insect bites, infections and similar conditions.

The first official report of its use by a doctor was in the Medicinal Journal of Australia in 1930 where a Sydney surgeon wrote of its wound healing and antiseptic properties.

During World War II, tea tree oil was added into machine "cutting" oils in munitions factories in Australia. This is said to have greatly reduced the number of infections due to abrasions on the hands of workers caused by the metal filings and turnings (slivers).

The Many Uses of Tea Tree Oil

Tea tree essential oil is considered to be both antiseptic (able to destroy bacteria capable of causing infection) and an antimicrobial (may destroy or prevent growth of microbes which are any tiny living things including bacteria, fungi, parasites and viruses). It is used medicinally in the treatment of many conditions, the most common being prevention or treatment of acne, fungal infections, yeast infections and a wide variety of skin conditions.

Tea tree oil works against bacteria and microbes in a similar way to disinfectants as it disrupts the cell membranes of destructive microorganisms, and disables the proteins within them, basically "de-activating" them so they cannot multiply and cause health problems. The main active constituents in tea tree oil are chemical compounds called terpinen-4-ol, alpha-terpineol, and linalool.

Using Tea Tree Oil for Prevention and Treatment

Where can you use Tea Tree Oil? Everywhere!

This booklet has been created as a handy guide that you can keep in your home, cottage, office or even your camper! You may be surprised how many ways a small bottle of tea tree oil can be used. If you are unsure about what kind of tea tree oil to look for, I recommend a 100% tea tree oil from a trusted supplier, such as Holista Health Canada (holista.com). You should be able to find this useful essential oil at your local natural health retailer, pharmacy or grocery store.

To further assist you in overcoming any health challenges you identify while reading this book, I have included nutritional supplement recommendations related to each condition or symptom. These are given in the interests of education and are not intended to prescribe, diagnose or as a substitute for the advice of your health practitioner.

In good health,

Dr. Joyce Tellier Johnson

P.S. If you have any additional ways to use
tea tree oil that I've missed, please let me know!
(email info@wnpharmaceuticals.com)

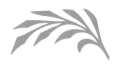

Head, Face, and Mouth

There are common health and cosmetic challenges that many people face (pardon the pun) related to hair, the scalp, facial skin, lips, mouth and teeth. In this section we look at some of the ways tea tree oil can help "at the top".

Acne *(Acne vulgaris)*

Acne is the most common skin problem in North America. One in 4 visitors to a dermatologist are there because they want help for this skin disorder that can present itself as pimples, blackheads, and whiteheads, or as inflammatory acne with accompanying pustules and cysts. Inflammation occurs when the follicle (pore) wall is broken and white blood cells move in to fight bacteria. Acne breakouts frequently appear on the face, but can also be seen on the chest, back and shoulders.

Acne generally begins at puberty because production of androgens, hormones related to sexual development, cause a change in the size and activity of the sweat and sebaceous glands.

Sebum is the semi-fluid oily mixture produced in your pores to keep the skin soft, flexible and waterproof.

Acne can be more than a cosmetic problem; it can cause emotional stress and can have a profound impact on self confidence. Tea tree oil is a naturally potent ally in the fight against acne.

Tea Tree Oil Remedy:

Tea tree oil is a natural antiseptic and antibiotic. It has been shown to lower the bacteria level and inflammation of acne as effectively as topical pharmaceutical medications without negative side effects such as dry skin, redness and peeling.

Dab a small amount of tea tree oil on blemishes three times per day. Alternatively, add 10 drops of tea tree oil to ¼ cup of warm water and wash blemished areas morning and night with a clean cotton ball or pad.

Supporting Research:

A clinical trial of 124 patients with acne vulgaris compared the use of tea tree oil to benzoyl peroxide over the course of 3 months. The tea tree oil product was significantly more effective at improving the acne condition and reducing the number of acne lesions. The tea tree oil was also better tolerated and had a reduced incidence of side effects such as dry skin, itchiness, and scaling skin.

Other Natural Remedies:

With tea tree oil as a topical support, acne may also be improved by using these natural supplements, taken internally.

Digestive enzymes
Essential Fatty Acids
Zinc
Chromium
Vitamin A
Vitamin B Complex
Vitamin E
Vitamin D
Selenium
Garlic

Canker Sores *(Aphthous stomatitis)*

Canker sores are a common condition. They are small, white swellings in the mouth that can develop into ulcers. Outbreaks vary from a single sore, two or three times a year, to an uninterrupted succession of multiple sores. These small, shallow mouth ulcers are painful and can be quite annoying. They appear either singly or in clusters on the roof of the mouth, on lips, gums, inner cheeks, tongue, and/or throat. The development of a canker sore may begin with a burning and tingling sensation. Canker sores typically heal without scarring within 1 to 3 weeks.

Tea Tree Oil Remedy:

Tea tree oil is NOT to be swallowed or ingested. It can be dabbed onto canker sores with a clean cotton swab. Do not use full strength for children. Dilute 5 to 10 drops in a quarter cup of warm water and dab onto the canker.

Other Natural Remedies:

With tea tree oil as topical support, canker sores may also be prevented or relieved by using these natural supplements, taken internally.

Acidophilus
L-Lysine
Vitamin B Complex
Multivitamin
Vitamin C with Bioflavonoids
Quercetin
Deglycyrrhizinated licorice (DGL)
Zinc lozenges

Chapped Lips

Dry, cracked lips can be caused by a dry environment, excessive licking or reaction to irritants in cosmetics or skin treatments. Chapped lips can be painful and unattractive and can interfere with basic day-to-day activities such as eating, talking and kissing!

Tea Tree Oil Remedy:

Add 5 drops of tea tree oil to your favorite lip balm or moisturizing cream. Apply to your lips as necessary, several times a day.

Other Natural Remedies:

Increase water intake
Essential fatty acids (Omega-3s, Evening Primrose Oil)

Cold Sores *(Herpes Simplex Virus 1)*

Cold sores, also called "fever blisters," are the result of chronic, recurrent viral infections caused by the herpes simplex virus 1 (HSV-1), which is related to the virus that causes genital herpes. "Herpes" is from the Greek "to creep" and the word was used by Herodotus in 100 BC to describe fever blisters.

Cold sores typically appear on the lips, or skin near the mouth, as single or multiple small bumps filled with fluid, within three to ten days after exposure to the herpes virus. They can last up to, or longer than, three weeks. Cold sores can spread and grow and are painful, itchy and irritating. Unfortunately, the virus remains permanently in the body, which is why some people are prone to frequent outbreaks. It is estimated that 80 percent of the population have been exposed to herpes simplex 1 and have antibodies against it. Strengthening immunity is important to preventing outbreaks.

Tea Tree Oil Remedy:

Tea tree oil can speed healing of cold sores. Apply a few drops on a cotton swab as soon as you feel the tenderness and itching that usually precede a cold sore. If the cold sore is already in full "bloom" apply a few drops of tea tree oil to the infected area twice a day.

Supporting Research:

A randomized, placebo-controlled study in 20 patients with cold sores (herpes labialis) investigated the effectiveness of a tea tree oil product and reported that it had benefits over the placebo. An in vitro study has also demonstrated the activity of tea tree oil against the herpes simplex viruses 1 and 2.

Other Natural Remedies:

Cold sores, and other viral infections, are most likely to occur when the immune system is weak or compromised. Strengthen your immunity and, with tea tree oil as topical support, use these natural supplements, taken internally, for long term health benefits.

L-Lysine
Vitamin B Complex
Acidophilus
Garlic
Vitamin C with Bioflavonoids
Vitamin A
Zinc

Common Cold (Rhinovirus)

Affecting the upper respiratory tract, the common cold is caused by a virus. Contrary to popular belief, cold weather and being exposed to drafts or temperature changes do NOT cause colds. Cold viruses survive better in colder temperatures, so they tend to thrive in the fall and winter months. Cold sufferers experience symptoms such as head congestion, runny nose, sore throat, sneezing, coughing, headache, and watery eyes. The majority of colds resolve on their own within 7 to 10 days, but occasionally they can lead to more serious illnesses involving the lungs (bronchitis, pneumonia), the ears (middle ear infections), and the sinuses.

Add 5 to 10 drops of tea tree oil to 4 cups of very hot water in a pot. Make a "steamer" by draping a towel over your head and over the pot. Inhale the steam. At night add 10 drops of tea tree oil to your vaporizer. You can also rub a drop on under your nose and on each temple. Eucalyptus Oil is another soothing oil for steam inhalation to clear breathing passages.

Other Natural Remedies:

With tea tree oil as topical support, help your body prevent or shorten the duration of colds by using these natural supplements, taken internally.

> Cold-A-Tak™ (concentrated Echinacea formula)
> E+3 (a supplement with Vitamin E, Selenium,
>   Vitamin A, and Vitamin C)
> Zinc/Zinc Lozenges
> Vitamin C with Bioflavonoids
> Garlic
> Maitake Extract
> Multivitamin and Mineralz

Dandruff

Dandruff is a common condition of the scalp that occurs when dead skin is shed or sloughed off. The result of this is annoying, often itchy, white flakes. Dandruff is typically more common in oily, rather than dry skin and is a result of skin cells renewing themselves. Everyone produces and sheds skin cells at different rates. New research shows that severe cases of dandruff may be caused by an overgrowth of a yeast called Pityrosporum ovale, that naturally resides on the skin.

Tea Tree Oil Remedy:

Add 20 drops of tea tree oil into your shampoo in the bottle and mix; use daily or alternate with another shampoo. Or use 3 drops of tea tree oil mixed with your shampoo in your hand to wash your hair. Rubbing a few drops of tea tree oil directly into the scalp may help unblock the hair follicles.

Supporting Research:

A 4-week trial in 126 patients with dandruff reported that a 5% tea tree oil product was more effective than the placebo and was well tolerated.

Other Natural Remedies:

Preventing or treating dandruff and other skin/scalp conditions can be easier if you maintain a healthy balance of nutrients. The following supplements can improve scalp and hair health.

Essential Fatty Acids
Kelp
Selenium
Vitamin B Complex
Vitamin B6
Vitamin B12
Vitamin E

Zinc
Vitamin A
Vitamin C with Bioflavonoids

Dental Care

The mouth is a breeding ground for bacteria. It is warm, moist and full of nooks and crannies where bacteria can hide, producing bad breath, promoting gum disease and tooth decay. Sore throats, canker sores and mouth ulcers are all too common.

Tea tree oil is NOT to be swallowed, so any oral use must be approached with care. Although some natural health practitioners recommend adding tea tree oil to your toothbrush, mouthwash or rinsing with it, I suggest using a commercial tea tree oil toothpaste or mouthwash rather than risking ingestion of too much of this potent oil.

Other Natural Remedies:

Brushing the teeth regularly and flossing can do a lot for mouth health, as can regular rinsing with hot water and salt, or a natural mouthwash. A balance of good nutrition can include immune builders such as Vitamin C and L-Lysine, and a good echinacea and zinc lozenge can improve a sore throat.

Ear Infections/Earaches

Approximately 75 percent of all children suffer from ear infections by the age of three. There are two types of ear infections that doctors encounter in their practices, *otitis externa* and *otitis media.* Swimmer's ear, also known as *otitis externa,* affects the outer ear and can include symptoms such as slight fever, discharge, and pain. A middle ear infection, *otitis media,* is very common in infants and children, and is an infection located behind the eardrum. This is where the small bones of the ear are located. If a bacteria or virus invades this region, inflammation and fluid build up, giving the sensation of pressure. Symptoms include earache, high fever, sharp, throbbing pain, and the feeling of fullness in the ear.

Tea Tree Oil Remedy:

For *otitis externa,* mix 5 drops of tea tree oil in 1/4 cup of warm olive oil. Drop a small amount gently into the ear, tilting the head to one side for a minute. Use small cotton ball or swab, gently, to absorb the oil. Repeat until improved.

Other Natural Remedies:

Prevention is important and a strong immune system is your best protection against infections. The following supplements support immunity and fight infections:

> Vitamin C with Bioflavonoids
> Zinc
> Vitamin B Complex
> Vitamin E
> Echinacea

Gum Disease *(Gingivitis)*

Gingivitis is a condition of the periodontal disease (pyorrhea) group. It is inflammation of the gums and is the early stage of periodontal disease. The main cause of gingivitis is poor hygiene characterized by plaque—deposits of bacteria, mucus, and food particles stuck to the teeth.

Tea Tree Oil Remedy:

As mentioned above, tea tree oil is NOT to be swallowed. Use a natural, commercial tea tree oil toothpaste or mouthwash rather than risking ingestion of too much of this potent oil.

Other Natural Remedies:

Brushing the teeth regularly and flossing can do a lot for mouth health, as can regular rinsing with hot water and salt or a natural mouthwash. The following nutrient supplements can also improve gum health:

Coenzyme Q10
Vitamin C with Bioflavonoids
Calcium and Magnesium
Zinc
Vitamin B Complex
Grape Seed Extract
Vitamin A
Vitamin E
Lactobacillus rinse

Head Lice/Scabies

Scabies is a parasitic disease of itch mites that burrow under the skin and lay eggs, causing a persistent, itchy rash. Lice, on the other hand, live on an individual or in the clothing that they wear. Scabies mites are transmitted from person to person, usually from prolonged contact whereas lice are transmitted from person to person and also from bedding and clothing.

Scabies is characterized by intense itching, skin burrows, and occasionally secondary infections with the most severe itching occurring at bedtime. The lesions and burrows are seen in the finger webs, wrists, beltline, groin, areola in females, and lower buttocks.

Lice may produce tiny black specks in the patients' undergarments and nits may be seen at the base of the hair shafts. Mild excoriations may be seen from scratching.

Tea Tree Oil Remedy:

For head lice, add 5 drops of Tea Tree Oil to 1 ounce of shampoo. (Or simply buy Holista Tea Tree Oil Shampoo). Massage into hair, leave on for 10 minutes, rinse; repeat once a day until eggs and lice are gone. This shampoo can also be used on the other areas affected by lice or scabies. Tea tree oil may be applied directly, twice a day, to an area affected by scabies, but it could cause irritation in people with sensitive skin. Consult a medical practitioner if an improvement is not seen within 10 days.

Supporting Research:

In test tube studies, topical application of tea tree oil was very effective against head lice with 93 percent of lice and 83 percent of eggs destroyed.

Other Natural Remedies:

Vitamin A
Garlic
Kelp
Zinc
Evening Primrose Oil (scabies)

Oral Thrush

Thrush is a fungal infection of the mouth characterized by creamy-white patches which form on the tongue and mucous membranes. Scraping the patches off can cause bleeding. Oral thrush is most commonly seen in infants or those individuals with compromised immune systems.

Tea Tree Oil Remedy:

I do not recommend gargling or other oral uses of tea tree oil, except if you use a natural, commercially prepared rinse or mouthwash. You may get relief by steaming over a pot of hot water with 5 to 10 drops of tea tree oil added.

Other Natural Remedies:

Acidophilus
Garlic
Vitamin B Complex

Vitamin C with Bioflavonoids
Vitamin E
Zinc
Essential Fatty Acids
Vitamin A
Cold-A-Tak™

Sinusitis

Sinusitis is an inflammation of the nasal sinuses. The most common cause of sinusitis is a viral upper respiratory infection, although bacteria, fungi, and allergic reactions may also be responsible. Any factor that creates swelling of the nasal tissues, resulting in obstruction and the lack of proper drainage of the area, will often lead to a sinus infection. Chronic sinusitis is most common in people with allergies, and dental infections account for 25 percent of chronic maxillary sinusitis. Swimming and diving, and injury to the area (especially a broken nose affecting the frontal sinuses) are other precipitating factors.

Tea Tree Oil Remedy:

Add 5 to 10 drops of tea tree oil to a pot of heated water. Drape a towel over your head. Lean over the pot and inhale gently. At night, add 10 drops to a vaporizer.

Other Natural Remedies:

Sinusitis may respond to the following dietary supplements due to their anti-bacterial, anti-inflammatory, or antioxidant action.

Acidophilus
Bee pollen
Flaxseed oil
Multivitamin and Mineral
Quercetin
Bromelain
Vitamin C with Bioflavonoids
Vitamin B Complex
Vitamin A
Zinc
Coenzyme Q10

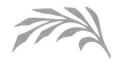

Throat, Chest, and Body

Some of the tips in section 1 will also apply to these parts of the body, but there are other ways tea tree oil can improve your mobility, flexibility, breathing, and immunity.

Arthritis (Osteoarthritis and Rheumatoid Arthritis)

Arthritis means inflammation of one or more joints. Osteoarthritis (OA) is the degeneration and loss of cartilage in the joints, with accompanying stiffness and pain. OA is the most common form of arthritis and can affect all the joints, but has special affinity for the weight-bearing joints (knees, hip, spine). It is seen in both men and women. In men it usually occurs before they are 45 years old, and in women after 45 to 55 years old. OA is very common and may have hereditary factors, but factors such as poor diet, trauma, and repetitive forceful stress to a joint, seem to precipitate arthritic conditions.

Rheumatoid arthritis (RA) is a chronic form of arthritis that can lead to destruction of the bone and cartilage resulting in characteristic deformities. It can appear in many forms: from a mild short-lasting illness that causes little damage, to a severe progressive disease causing significant joint destruction. Rheumatoid arthritis (RA) occurs in about 1 percent of the population, about three times as often in women as in men. RA usually occurs between the ages of 35 to 50 and has a genetic association.

Tea Tree Oil Remedy:

For joint swelling and pain due to arthritis, add 10 drops of tea tree oil to 2 ounces of jojoba or grapeseed oil and massage affected areas 2 to 3 times a day. Tea tree oil appears to be able to penetrate the joint and desensitize irritated nerve endings.

Other Natural Remedies:

Osteoarthritis:
Multivitamin and Mineral
Essential fatty acids—Omega-3s from fish or flaxseed
Glucosamine sulfate
Chondroitin sulfate
MSM
Celadrin®
S-Adenosyl-L-methionine (SAMe)
Turmeric
Bromelain

Rheumatoid Arthritis:
Multivitamin and Mineral
Betaine HCl
Vitamin E

Selenium
Bromelain
Vitamin C
Omega 3
EPO
Quercetin
Celadrin®

Bladder Infection *(Cystitis)*

Bladder infections are acute inflammations/infections of the urinary bladder. They are very common and occur in females 10 times more often than in males, except as infants when both sexes are equally affected. Symptoms include painful urination or a feeling that you have to urinate but cannot. More severe bladder infections can cause back pain and fever. Cranberry extract and blueberry extract capsules are an excellent oral supplement for urinary tract infections.

Tea Tree Oil Remedy:

It is important to keep the urethra and genital area clean to prevent infections and shorten their duration. Add 3 drops of tea tree oil to 4 ounces of purified or distilled water and wash genital area thoroughly. Put 10 drops of tea tree oil into hot bath water for a soothing soak.

Other Natural Remedies:

Cranberry or Blueberry concentrated extracts
Uva Ursi herbal extract *(Arctostaphylos uva ursi)*
Acidophilus and Bifidus

Multivitamin and Mineral
B complex
Vitamin C with Bioflavonoids
Garlic
Zinc

Bronchitis

Bronchitis is an infection of the trachea (windpipe) and bronchioles ("branches") that usually follows an upper respiratory infection like a cold or cough. Bronchitis is most common in the winter. Other factors involved in developing bronchitis include air pollution, chronic sinusitis, as well as irritating fumes (acute irritative bronchitis), such as ammonia, smoke, chlorine and others.

Tea Tree Oil Remedy:

Add 3 drops of tea tree oil to a warm, damp cloth; apply to chest or add 10 drops of tea tree oil to a hot bath and soak.

Other Natural Remedies:

Vitamin C
Vitamin A
Echinacea (clinically researched Cold-A-Tak™)
Zinc
Vitamin B Complex
Quercetin
Coenzyme Q10
MSM
Greens Powder

Multivitamin and Mineral
N-Acetylcysteine (NAC)

Bruises

A bruise is formed when tissues below the skin are injured due to physical trauma. The skin remains intact, but the capillaries carrying blood below the surface are broken and blood is able to drain into surrounding tissue. People who do not consume enough fresh, uncooked foods to provide the body with needed nutrients are more likely to bruise easily.

Tea Tree Oil Remedy:

Apply ice if swelling occurs. Mix 5 drops of tea tree oil into an arnica or comfrey salve. Apply daily as needed.

Other Natural Remedies:
Multivitamin and Mineral
Vitamin C with Bioflavonoids
Alfalfa
Vitamin E
Vitamin B Complex
Vitamin D
Iron (if anemic)
Coenzyme Q10

Burns

The skin is the body's largest organ, which makes a serious burn one of the most traumatic injuries the body can sustain. First-degree burns involve the surface of the skin. They can cause mild pain, redness, dry skin, and swelling. No blisters form and healing usually occurs without scarring in 2 to 3 days. An example would be a typical sunburn.

Second-degree burns involve deeper layers of the skin, including the upper level of the dermis. Skin functions are lost, blisters form, pain and swelling are present and healing can take a week to 10 days with possible scarring.

Third-degree burns include destruction of both the epidermis and dermis. Skin functions are lost, there is no pain in the immediate area of the burn due to destruction of nerve endings, but there may be extreme pain in surrounding tissue. Regeneration of the skin following a third-degree burn is slow and may require skin grafts, leaving an obvious scar.

Tea Tree Oil Remedy:

Tea tree oil can help speed healing of a minor, first-degree, burn. Immediately wash the area with ice water, and apply a few drops of tea tree oil to the burned area. Repeat 3 to 4 times daily. For a healing salve, mix 20 drops of tea tree oil with 3 ounces raw unpasteurized honey and 1/2 teaspoon triple strength grapefruit seed extract.

Other Natural Remedies:

Topically:
Calendula officinalis
Aloe vera gel

Orally:
Potassium
Vitamin A
Vitamin B Complex
Vitamin C with Bioflavonoids
Vitamin E
Zinc
Essential Fatty Acids
Calcium and Magnesium with D
Coenzyme Q10

Coughs

Congestion in the lungs, from viral infections or irritation, can result in coughing, with or without excess mucous and phlegm.

Tea Tree Oil Remedy:

Add 6 to 8 drops of tea tree oil to 4 to 6 cups warm water. Drape a towel over your head and lean over warm water for 10 minutes and gently inhale the vapours. At night you can add 10 drops tea tree oil to the water in a vaporizer and let it steam for 5 to 10 minutes.

Other Natural Remedies:

Natural cough syrups with horehound, wild
cherry, mullein, eucalyptus and honey.

Zinc lozenges

Cuts and Wounds

Tea Tree Oil Remedy:

Tea tree oil should not be applied directly into open cuts or
wounds, but a diluted mixture (10 drops of TTO in a cup of
warm water) may be applied as an antiseptic wash or on a cloth
bandage if the cut or wound is stitched or closed.

Other Natural Remedies:

Calendula

Vitamin E oil

Dermatitis/Eczema

Dermatitis is a general name given to any inflammation of the
skin. Often the terms dermatitis and eczema are used inter-
changeably. Eczema can be caused by a number of things such
as stress, fatigue, and nutrient deficiency, which all play a role
in allowing environmental or internal irritants to cause skin
discomfort and these various skin conditions.

Tea Tree Oil Remedy:

Tea tree oil is a natural antiseptic and antibiotic. It can lower
the bacteria level on the skin without negative side effects such
as dry skin, redness and peeling. However, depending upon the

severity of the condition, you will want to test a small patch of skin before using tea tree oil broadly, to determine sensitivity.

Dab a small amount of tea tree oil on an affected area. If no irritation occurs repeat on other areas. You can also add 10 drops of tea tree oil to 1/4 cup of warm water and wash affected areas morning and night with a clean 100% cotton ball or pad, then pat until very dry.

Other Natural Remedies:
    Betaine HCl
    MSM
    Vitamin B Complex
    Omega-3
    Evening Primrose Oil
    Kelp
    Vitamin C with Bioflavonoids
    Vitamin E
    Zinc
    Acidophilus
    Vitamin A
    Vitamin D
    B Complex
    Quercetin
    Selenium
    Zinc oxide topically with Vitamin E

Hemorrhoids

Hemorrhoids are swollen veins (varicose) veins around the anus and in the rectum that may protrude from the anus. If the hemorrhoids are located inside the anal canal, they are called internal hemorrhoids. If located at the anal opening, they are called external hemorrhoids.

Factors that increase your risk of hemorrhoid formation include:

heredity
pregnancy
sedentary lifestyle
straining at stool: chronic constipation
standing for long periods of time
sitting on hard, cold surfaces
liver stagnancy or disease (cirrhosis)
benign prostatic hypertrophy

Tea Tree Oil Remedy:

Apply a mixture of tea tree oil (about 5 drops) and a natural oil like olive or almond oil, to the affected area twice daily.

Other Natural Remedies:

Vitamin C with Bioflavonoids
Flaxseed oil
Ground Flaxseed powder
Psyllium seed powder
Calcium and Magnesium
Vitamin E
Vitamin B Complex

Genital Herpes *(Herpes Simplex Virus 2)*

Genital herpes is the most common sexually transmitted disease. On average, one out of every five persons over the age of twelve have it, although more than half never develop serious symptoms. Systemic symptoms also include fever, muscle pain, general malaise and headaches. Genital complaints include pain (can be severe), itching, vaginal and urethral discharge. In women, most initial infections involve the cervix and urethra. Patients who already have cold sores caused by HSV-1 may have a less intense primary attack of genital herpes. Recurrences of genital herpes are common, usually within 1-4 months of the first outbreak; the average number of recurrences experienced is 4-7 episodes a year.

Tea Tree Oil Remedy:

Mix 2 drops of tea tree oil with the contents of 1 capsule of natural source Vitamin E and apply to herpes lesions twice daily. Discontinue use if irritation occurs. You can also add 10 drops of tea tree oil to bath water or a Sitz bath.

Supporting Research:

An in vitro study has demonstrated activity of tea tree oil against the herpes simplex viruses 1 and 2.

Other Natural Remedies:

The following supplements can help improve immunity and reduce frequency or severity of HSV 1 and 2 attacks.

Orally:
L-Lysine
Vitamin C with Bioflavonoids
Vitamin A
Vitamin B Complex
Zinc
Acidophilus
Essential Fatty Acids
Garlic
Vitamin E

Topically:
Licorice Root *(Glycyrrhiza)*
Topical Vitamin E and Zinc

Hives (Urticaria)

Hives is a skin condition characterized by sudden outbreaks of red, itchy welts. Hives are relatively common, with about 15–20 percent of the population having experienced them. Although seen in all ages, hives seem to be more prevalent among young adults (post-adolescence until 30 years old). The reaction is basically an allergic response. Hives usually resolve within a few hours to a couple of days, but in rare cases they become chronic and may last for six weeks or more.

Tea Tree Oil Remedy:

Add 4 drops of tea tree oil to 2 ounces of witch hazel. Massage affected area.

Other Natural Remedies:

Acidophilus
Flaxseed oil
Evening Primrose Oil
Garlic
Multivitamin and Mineral
Vitamin B Complex
Vitamin C with Bioflavonoids
Quercetin
Vitamin E
Vitamin D

Jock Itch

Fungal infections of the skin occur most commonly in places that are moist and where one skin surface is in contact with another. Jock itch is a fungal infection of the skin in the groin area.

Tea Tree Oil Remedy:

Apply several times per day to the affected area either full strength or diluted with distilled water or cold-pressed vegetable oil.

Other Natural Remedies:

Acidophilus
Garlic
Vitamin B Complex
Vitamin C with Bioflavonoids
Vitamin E

Zinc
Essential Fatty Acids
Vitamin A

Laryngitis

Laryngitis is an inflammation of the larynx. Most laryngitis is caused by microorganisms, viral and bacterial (especially streptococcus). It can also occur concurrently with other infections such as urinary tract infections and lung infections. Other causes include voice overuse, allergic reactions, and inhaling irritating substances (e.g. smoking).

Tea Tree Oil Remedy:

I do not recommend gargling with tea tree oil, except if you use a natural, commercially prepared rinse or mouthwash. You may get relief by steaming over a pot of hot water with 5–10 drops of tea tree oil added.

Other Natural Remedies:
Vitamin C
Vitamin A
Zinc, Zinc Lozenges

Muscle Pain

Over-exertion or sudden straining can cause muscles to become inflamed and tender. Some of the healing power of tea tree oil is apparently able to penetrate the skin and ease sore muscles.

Tea Tree Oil Remedy:

Mix 5 drops of tea tree oil with 1 ounce of grapeseed oil. Massage well. You can also add 10 drops to bath water and soak.

Other Natural Remedies:

Creatine
L-Glutamine
Calcium/Magnesium supplements

Psoriasis

Psoriasis is one of the most common chronic skin diseases. Most patients experience the onset before age 20. Psoriasis appears as patches of skin on the legs, knees, arms, elbows, scalp, ears, and back that are red to brown in coloured and covered with silvery-white scales. There seems to be a genetic tendency, as 30 percent of patients have a family history that includes psoriasis. The exact cause is unknown.

Tea Tree Oil Remedy:

Tea tree oil is a natural antiseptic and antibiotic. It can lower the bacteria level on the skin without negative side effects such as dry skin, redness and peeling. However, depending upon the severity of the psoriasis, you will want to test a small patch of skin before using tea tree oil broadly, to determine sensitivity.

Dab a small amount of tea tree oil on an affected area. If no irritation occurs repeat on other areas. You can also add 10 drops of tea tree oil to 1/4 cup of warm water and wash affected areas morning and night with a clean cotton ball or pad, then pat until very dry.

Other Natural Remedies:
Multivitamin and Mineral
Omega-3
Flaxseed Oil
Evening Primrose Oil
Zinc
Vitamin A
Chromium
Evening Primrose Oil
Vitamin E
Vitamin D
Vitamin B Complex
Vitamin C with Bioflavonoids
MSM
Selenium
Milk Thistle

Ringworm

Ringworm, also known as a tinea infection, is a fungal infection that occurs on the skin or scalp. It is characterized by the appearance of small red spots that increase in size to approximately 1/4 inch in diameter. Ringworm is an infection that can be extremely itchy.

Tea Tree Oil Remedy:

Ringworm is not a worm but a fungus. Apply tea tree oil to affected areas, full strength, twice daily. Stop use if irritation occurs.

Other Natural Remedies:

    Acidophilus
    Garlic
    Vitamin B Complex
    Vitamin C with Bioflavonoids
    Vitamin E
    Zinc
    Essential Fatty Acids
    Vitamin A

Sore Throat

One of the most common health complaints, sore throats can vary from raw, burning, and scratching feeling, to a sense of fullness and discomfort when swallowing. Viral infections are the most common culprits when it comes to sore throats which often go hand-in-hand with the common cold. However, sore throats can also be caused by substances that irritate the back of the throat.

Tea Tree Oil Remedy:

I do not recommend gargling with tea tree oil, except if you use a natural, commercially prepared rinse or mouthwash. You may get relief by steaming over a pot of hot water with 5–10 drops of tea tree oil added. A hot water and salt gargle is also effective.

Other Natural Remedies:
Acidophilus
Bee Propolis
Garlic
Maitake Extract
Multivitamin and Mineral
Vitamin A
Vitamin C with Bioflavonoids
Vitamin E
Zinc lozenges
Echinacea (Cold-A-Tak™)

Vaginitis

Vaginitis is an infection of the vaginal tract that causes inflammation of the vaginal lining. Although vaginitis can be caused by a sexually transmitted infectious micro-organism, it is more typically due to a disturbance in the delicate ecology of the vagina that allows organisms normally found in a healthy vagina to overgrow and produce an infection.

Tea Tree Oil Remedy:

Apply a few drops of the oil on a tampon, or mix with water and use it as a douche. Topical tea tree oil cream can also be used.

Supporting Research:

The World Health Organization in 2003 stated that clinical data supported the use of tea tree oil for vaginitis and cervicitis. A study found that intravaginal application of tampons soaked in a diluted tea tree oil solution successfully healed vaginitis and cervicitis in 130 patients with a Trichomonas vaginalis infection. Vaginal "suppositories", containing 0.2 g tea tree essential oil, inserted nightly eradicated symptoms and burning in women with Candida albicans vaginitis after 30 days in 86 percent of women, with a full 75 percent free of infection.

Other Natural Remedies:

Orally:
Acidophilus
Multivitamin and Mineral
Garlic
Essential Fatty Acids
Vitamin B Complex
E+3 (a supplement with Vitamin E, Selenium, Vitamin A, and Vitamin C)
Vitamin C with Bioflavonoids
Vitamin D
Zinc
Echinacea (Cold-A-Tak™)

Topically:
Aloe vera
Calendula and Vitamin A suppositories

Warts

Warts are small growths caused by human papilloma viruses (HPV). Although warts may occur at any age, they are most common in older children and are rarely seen in the elderly. Warts can be found anywhere in the body, but are most commonly found on the hands, fingers, elbows, forearms, knees, faces, and skin around the nails.

Tea Tree Oil Remedy:

Apply full strength tea tree oil to wart. It may take several weeks for wart to dissolve, depending upon conditions.

Other Natural Remedies:

Vitamin B Complex
Vitamin A
Vitamin E
Vitamin C with Bioflavonoids
MSM
Zinc
Multivitamin and Mineral

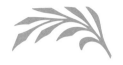

Legs and Feet

They carry us around all day and are often ignored when it comes to tender loving care, but our legs and feet need love too! Tea tree oil's popularity doesn't stop at athlete's foot, although it has been one of the most common uses of this potent natural ally.

Athlete's Foot *(Tinea pedis)*

Athlete's foot is a tinea infection, one that thrives in an environment that is warm and moist. The fungus lives off the dead skin cells and calluses of the feet, especially between the toes. It is very common in gyms and in swimming pools and locker rooms. Symptoms can range from simple peeling of skin, to deep cracking and severe itching and inflammation.

Tea Tree Oil Remedy:

Soak feet in foot bath with 20 drops of tea tree oil for fifteen minutes three times daily (or as often as possible). Dry feet off thoroughly and apply tea tree oil, full strength, on affected areas.

Supporting Research:

In a double-blind, randomized trial of 158 patients with athlete's foot, the effectiveness of two strengths of tea tree oil (25% and 50%) were compared. After applying the tea tree oil twice daily for four weeks, the authors concluded that both strengths were effective. The 25% tea tree oil preparation had fewer complications and was more highly recommended by the authors of the study.

Another double-blind, randomized trial treated 104 patients with athlete's foot using 10% tea tree oil cream compared to 1 percent tolnaftate or placebo creams. This study showed that the tolnaftate caused the greatest reduction in the fungal infection, over tea tree oil and placebo creams, however tea tree oil cream was *as* effective at reducing symptoms.

Other Natural Remedies:

Acidophilus
Garlic
Vitamin B Complex
Vitamin C with Bioflavonoids
Zinc
Essential Fatty Acids
Vitamin A
Vitamin E

Blisters

A blister is rather like a burn from friction on the skin and it can be easily infected. Keep the area clean and treat with tea tree oil. Cover with a bandage if necessary.

Tea Tree Oil Remedy:

Apply tea tree oil full strength to the affected area.

Corns and Calluses

Corns and calluses are overgrowths of skin tissue (hyperkeratosis) that eventually thicken and harden. Calluses occur most commonly on areas that incur a lot of friction such as the soles of the feet and the hands. Corns are skin overgrowths that are cone-shaped and most often form between the toes. These growths can cause inflammation and pain.

Tea Tree Oil Remedy:

Add 3 drops of tea tree oil to 1 teaspoon grapeseed, apricot, olive, almond or avocado oil. Massage into the corn or callus well, or soak the feet in a mixture of 10 drops tea tree oil, 1/2 ounce grapeseed, apricot, olive, almond or avocado oil for 5 minutes, twice daily. Once the corn or calluses have become soft, remove with tweezers and apply a few drops of tea tree oil, then cover with bandage.

Other Natural Remedies:

Topical Vitamin E oil

Gout

Gout is a common type of arthritis which typically begins in the first joint of the big toe. It is a disorder of protein metabolism leading to an increased concentration of uric acid. In gout, uric acid crystals (monosodium urate) deposit in joints, tendons, kidneys, and other tissues, causing considerable inflammation and damage. Kidney involvement may lead to kidney failure. Gout occurs more commonly in men.

Tea Tree Oil Remedy:

For joint swelling caused by gout, mix 5 drops of tea tree oil with 2 ounces of jojoba or grapeseed oil and massage into the affected area 2–3 times a day.

Other Natural Remedies:

Multivitamin and Mineral
Omega-3
Vitamin E
Folic Acid
Bromelain
Devil's Claw
Quercetin
Vitamin B Complex
Vitamin C with Bioflavonoids
Kelp or alfalfa
Grape seed extract
Zinc
Calcium and Magnesium
Glucosamine

Chondroitin
Celadrin® (oral or topical applications are available)
MSM

Leg Ulcers

When the legs experience poor circulation, blood flow is restricted, the skin tissue can erode and ulcers form. Due to the poor circulation, healing times of leg ulcers can be quite slow. Leg ulcers tend to occur in individuals with poor circulation such as in diabetic patients.

Tea Tree Oil Remedy:

Apply 8 drops of tea tree oil to 3 cups of warm water or add 5 drops of tea tree oil to 1 ounce grapeseed oil. Shake well and massage into area.

Other Natural Remedies:

Coenzyme Q10
Garlic
Grape seed extract
Vitamin C with Bioflavonoids
Vitamin E
Flaxseed oil
Multivitamin and Mineral
Vitamin B Complex
Zinc
Echinacea

Nail Infections *(Paronychia and Onychomycosis)*

Paronychia is an infection that develops along the edge of the fingernail or toenail. Fungal infections under the nails can cause the nail to rise off the nail bed and cause swelling of the nail bed and discolouration of the nail. *Onychomycosis* is a fungal infection of the nail that results in thickening, roughness, and splitting of the nails. It can lead to a complete destruction of the nail. Both these infections may be improved with the use of tea tree oil.

Tea Tree Oil Remedy:

Pour 2–3 drops of tea tree oil directly to nail and tissue surroundings. Repeat every morning and night. These infections can be persistent so you must be as well. Increase frequency of application when you can.

Supporting Research:

In a randomized, controlled trial of 117 patients suffering from *onychomycosis* compared the effectiveness of tea tree oil to a topical medication (1% clotrimazole cream) over a 6 month period. Improvements in both groups were comparable as was the cost of the treatments. A second randomized, double-blind, placebo-controlled trial compared the combination cream containing tea tree oil (5% tea tree oil and 2% butenafine hydrochloride) to a placebo. Over the 16-week trial observing 60 patients with *onychomycosis*, 80 percent of those who used the tea tree oil preparation were cured compared to no cures at all in the placebo group.

Other Natural Remedies:

   Acidophilus
   Garlic
   Vitamin B Complex
   Vitamin C with Bioflavonoids
   Vitamin E
   Zinc
   Essential Fatty Acids
   Vitamin A
   Silica
   Calcium and Magnesium with Vitamin D

Plantar Warts

Plantar warts are found on the soles of the feet and also on the underside of the toes. They are characterized by white raised growths that resemble calluses and interrupt the natural 'footprint.' They can be tender to touch and may bleed if scraped or trimmed.

Tea Tree Oil Remedy:

Apply tea tree oil full strength to affected area 2–3 times daily.

Other Natural Remedies:

   Vitamin B Complex
   Vitamin A
   Vitamin E
   Vitamin C with Bioflavonoids
   MSM
   Zinc

Multivitamin and Mineral

Topical:

Tape occlusion technique (Also called the "Red Green Approach"). Apply duct tape over the wart for approximately two months changing periodically.

Summary

More than any other single "herb," the essential oil of the tea tree has gathered a following of dedicated users who continue to find ways to use this simple product to enhance their lives or help prevent illness and infections. I haven't touched on the ways this unique oil can be added to household products for cleaning and disinfecting—but that doesn't mean you can't look into those as well.

There are many different concentrations of tea tree oils and lotions available. There are tea tree oil shampoos and conditioners. There is everything from tea tree oil lip balm to tea tree oil toothpaste. Enjoy trying a variety of tea tree oil options for your family and your home.

One last word of warning: Do NOT use tea tree oil on your pets. It could be harmful to them and is NOT advised. Naturally trained veterinarians have products appropriate for your pet's good health.

Dr. Joyce Tellier Johnson

References

Altman, P. Australian tea tree oil. Aust. J. Pharm. 1988;69:276-78.

Balch PA. Prescription for Nutritional Healing. 4th ed. New York, NY: Penguin Books Limited; 2006.

Bassett IB, Pannowitz DL, Barnetson RS. A comparative study of tea-tree oil versus benzoylperoxide in the treatment of acne. Med J Aust. 1990;153(8): 455-458.

Belaiche P. Letter to the Editor. Phytotherapy Res. 2:157;1988.

Blackwell AL. Tea tree oil and anaerobic (bacterial) vaginosis. Lancet 337.8736(1991):300.

Brown D. Topical tea tree oil for onychomycosis. Quarterly Review of Natural Medicine. 1995;Spring:11.

Boon H, Smith M. The Complete Natural Medicine Guide to the 50 Most Common Medicinal Herbs. Toronto: The Institute of Naturopathic Medicine and Research (The Canadian College of Naturopathic Medicine); 2004.

Braun L, Cohen M. Herbs and Natural Supplements – An evidence-based guide. Elsevier Health Sciences; 2004.

Brown D. Tea tree oil for athlete's foot. Quarterly Review of Natural Medicine. 1993;Winter:15.

Buck DS, Nidorf DM, Addino JG. Comparison of two topical preparations for the treatment of onychomycosis: Melaleuca alternifolia (tea tree) oil and clotrimazole. J Fam Pract. 1994;38: 601-605.

Carson CF, Ashton L, Dry L, Smith DW, Riley TV. Melaleuca alternifolia (tea tree) oil gel (6%) for the treatment of recurrent herpes labialis. J Antimicrob Chemother. 2001;48(3):450-51.

Concha JM, Moore LS, Holloway WJ. 1998 William J. Stickel Bronze Award. Antifungal activity of Melaleuca alternifolia (tea tree) oil against various pathogenic organisms. J Am Podiatr Med Assoc 88.10(1998)489-92.

Cox SD et al. The mode of antimicrobial action of the essential oil of Melaleuca alternifolia (tea tree oil) J Appl Microbiol 88.1 (2000):170-75.

Gustafson JE et al. Effects of tea tree oil on Escherichia coli. Lett Appl Microbiol 26.3(1998):194-98.

Hammer, K. A., Carson, C. F. & Riley, T. V. Susceptibility of transient and commensal skin flora to the essential oil of Melaleuca alternifolia (tea tree oil). Am J Infect Control 24.3(1996):186-89.

Hammer, K. A., Carson, C. F. & Riley, T. V. In vitro activity of essential oils, in particular Melaleuca alternifolia (tea tree) oil and tea tree oil products, against Candida spp. J Antimicrob Chemother 42.5(1998):591-95.

Hammer, K. A., Carson, C. F. & Riley, T. V. In vitro activities of ketoconazole, econazole, miconazole, and Melaleuca alternifolia (tea tree) oil against Malassezia species. Antimicrobial Agents and Chemotherapy (2000) 44:467-469.

Jacobs MR, Hornfeldt CS. Melaleuca oil poisoning. J Toxicol Clin Toxicol 32.4(1994):461-64.

Prepubertal Gynecomastia Linked to Lavender and Tea Tree Oils. N Engl J Med (2007); 356:479-485.

Leung AY, Foster S. Encyclopedia of Common Natural Ingredients used in Food, Drugs, and Cosmetics. 2ne ed. Toronto, ON/New York, NY: John Wiley and Sons Inc; 1996.

Murray M. The healing power of herbs. 1995, Prima Health, USA.

Pizzorno L, Pizzorno J, Murray M. Natural Medicine Instructions for Patients. Elsevier Health Sciences; 2002.

Satchell AC, Saurajen A, Bell C, Barnetson RS. Treatment of interdigital tinea pedis with 25% and 50% tea tree oil solution: a randomized, placebo-controlled, blinded study. Australasian J Dermatol. 2002;43(3):175-178.

Satchell AC, Saurajen A, Bell C, Barnetson RS. Treatment of dandruff with 5% tea tree oil shampoo. J Am Acad Dermatol. 2002;47(6):852-855.

Schnitzler P, Schon K, Reichling J. Antiviral activity of Australian tea tree oil and eucalyptus oil against herpes simplex virus in cell culture. Pharmazie 56.4(2001):343-47.

Syed TA, Qureshi ZA, Ali SM, Ahmad S, Ahmad SA. Treatment of toenail onychomycosis with 2% butenafine and 5% Melaleuca alternifolia (tea tree) oil in cream. Trop Med Int Health. 1999;4(4):284-287.

Tisserand R, Balacs T. Essential Oil Safety: A Guide for Health Care Professionals. London: Churchill Livingstone; 1995.

Tong, M.M., Altman, P.M. and Barnetson, R. St.-C. Tea tree oil in the treatment of Tinea pedis. Australian J. Dermatology. 1992;33:145-149.

Tyler VE. Robbers JE. Tyler's Herbs of Choice. The Therapeutic Use of Phytomedicinals. Binghampton, NY: The Haworth Herbal Press; 2000.

Tyler VE. Tyler's Honest Herbal. 4th ed. Binghampton, NY: The Haworth Herbal Press; 2000.

Veal L. The potential effectiveness of essential oils as a treatment for headlice, Pediculus humanus capitis. Complement Ther Nurs Midwifery 2.4(1996):97-101.

Walton, SF, et al. Acaricidal Activity of Melaleuca alternifolia (Tea Tree) Oil. In Vitro Sensitivity of Sarcoptes scabiei var hominis to Terpinen-4-ol. Arch Dermatol. (2004)140:563-566.

Williams L, Home V.A. A comparative study of some essential oils for potential use in topical applications for the treatment of the yeast Candida albincans. Australian Journal of Medical Herbalism. 1995;7(3):57-62.